Created by BabyDreamers.net

Free Book Offer:

Get How to be a Super Mom For Free

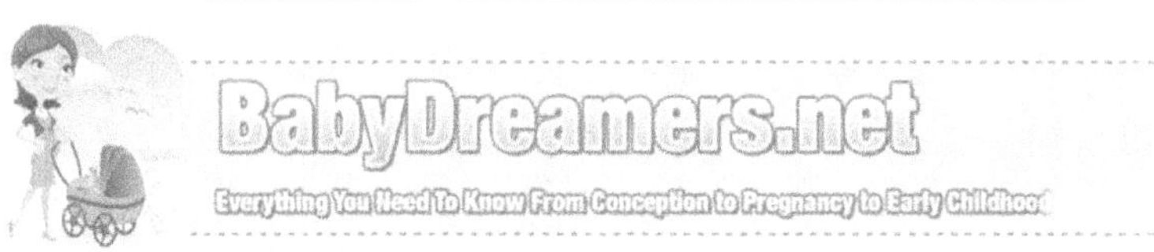

A Short Read is a type of book that is designed to be read in one quick sitting.

These no fluff books are perfect for people who want an overview about a subject in a short period of time.

Table of Contents

The Impact of Age on Fertility: What Every Woman Should Know

The Impact of Age on Fertility: What Every Woman Should Know

As women, it is essential for us to understand the relationship between age and fertility. It is a topic that can often be overlooked or misunderstood, but it plays a significant role in our ability to conceive and have a healthy pregnancy. In this article, we will explore the impact of age on fertility and provide important information that every woman should know.

Age is a crucial factor when it comes to fertility. As we age, our reproductive system undergoes natural changes that can affect our ability to conceive. It is important to be aware of these changes and how they can impact our chances of getting pregnant.

One of the key factors influenced by age is the quantity and quality of our eggs. As we get older, the number of eggs we have decreases, and the remaining eggs may not be as healthy or viable as they were in our younger years. This decline in egg quantity and quality can make it more challenging to conceive and increase the risk of pregnancy complications.

Another important aspect to consider is the impact of age on our menstrual cycle and reproductive hormones. As we age, our menstrual cycle may become irregular, and ovulation patterns may change. Additionally, the levels of reproductive hormones such as estrogen and progesterone may fluctuate, affecting our fertility.

It is also crucial to understand the role of Anti-Mullerian Hormone (AMH) in assessing ovarian reserve and its correlation with age-related fertility decline. Ovarian reserve testing can provide valuable insights into a woman's fertility potential and help predict her chances of conceiving.

For women who are trying to conceive at an older age, there are fertility treatments available, such as In Vitro Fertilization (IVF). IVF can help overcome age-related fertility challenges and increase the chances of pregnancy. Another option that has gained popularity is egg freezing, which allows women to preserve their fertility and increase their chances of conception in the future.

However, it is important to note that age can also bring increased risks and complications during pregnancy. Advanced maternal age is associated with a higher risk of miscarriage and birth defects, such as Down syndrome. Prenatal testing and screening play a crucial role in assessing these risks and making informed decisions about pregnancy.

Addressing the emotional aspects of fertility and age is equally important. Women may face emotional challenges when dealing with age-related infertility and the pressure to conceive. It is essential to seek support from support groups, counseling, and therapy to navigate this journey.

In conclusion, age has a significant impact on fertility. Understanding the relationship between age and fertility is crucial for every woman. By being aware of these factors, we can make informed decisions about our reproductive health and explore alternative paths to parenthood if needed.

Understanding Female Fertility

Female fertility is a complex and intricate process that involves various factors. To understand female fertility, it is important to have an overview of the female reproductive system and the factors that influence fertility, including age, hormonal balance, and overall health.

The female reproductive system consists of organs such as the ovaries, fallopian tubes, uterus, and cervix. The ovaries are responsible for producing eggs, also known as ova, which are released during ovulation. The fallopian tubes serve as a pathway for the eggs to travel from the ovaries to the uterus. The uterus, or womb, is where a fertilized egg implants and develops into a fetus. The cervix is the lower part of the uterus that connects to the vagina.

Age plays a significant role in female fertility. As women age, their fertility naturally declines. This is due to a decrease in the number and quality of eggs. Women are born with a finite number of eggs, and as they age, the quantity and quality of these eggs diminish. This decline in egg quantity and quality can make it more difficult for women to conceive and increase the risk of pregnancy complications.

Hormonal balance is another crucial factor in female fertility. Hormones such as estrogen and progesterone play a vital role in regulating the menstrual cycle and preparing the uterus for pregnancy. Any hormonal imbalances can disrupt the normal functioning of the reproductive system and affect fertility.

Overall health also plays a significant role in female fertility. Factors such as body weight, nutrition, exercise, and underlying medical conditions can impact a woman's ability to conceive. Maintaining a healthy lifestyle, including a balanced diet and regular exercise, can contribute to optimal fertility.

In conclusion, understanding female fertility involves comprehending the intricacies of the female reproductive system and the various factors that influence fertility. Age, hormonal balance, and overall health all play crucial roles in a woman's fertility journey. By understanding these factors, women can make informed decisions about their reproductive health and take proactive steps to optimize their fertility.

The Decline in Fertility with Age

The decline in fertility with age is a natural process that every woman should be aware of. As women age, there is a decrease in the number and quality of eggs, which can significantly impact their ability to conceive. This decline in egg quantity and quality is due to a natural aging process that affects the ovaries.

With age, a woman's ovarian reserve, which refers to the number of eggs she has remaining, gradually diminishes. This means that as a woman gets older, she has fewer eggs available for fertilization. Additionally, the quality of the remaining eggs may also decline, making it more difficult for them to successfully fertilize and implant in the uterus.

Along with the decrease in egg quantity and quality, there is also an increased risk of pregnancy complications as women age. These complications can include gestational diabetes, high blood pressure, and genetic disorders. The risk of miscarriage also increases with age, as does the incidence of birth defects such as Down syndrome and other chromosomal abnormalities.

It is important for women to understand the impact of age on fertility and the potential risks associated with trying to conceive at an older age. By being aware of these factors, women can make informed decisions about their reproductive health and consider alternative options if necessary.

Age and Egg Quantity

As women age, their egg quantity decreases, which can have significant implications on their chances of getting pregnant. A woman is born with a finite number of eggs, and as she gets older, the number of eggs in her ovaries gradually declines. This natural decline in egg quantity is known as ovarian reserve depletion.

The decrease in egg quantity can affect a woman's fertility because fewer eggs mean fewer opportunities for fertilization and pregnancy. Additionally, the quality of the remaining eggs may also diminish with age, making it more difficult for them to be successfully fertilized and develop into a healthy embryo.

Age-related decline in egg quantity is a key factor in the decreased fertility experienced by women as they get older. It is important for women to be aware of this decline and understand that their chances of conceiving naturally may decrease as they age. However, it is worth noting that every woman is unique, and fertility can vary from person to person.

There are various tests available to assess a woman's ovarian reserve and determine her egg quantity. These tests can provide valuable information about a woman's fertility potential and help her make informed decisions about family planning. It is recommended that women who are concerned about their fertility consult with a healthcare professional or fertility specialist to discuss their options and understand the implications of age-related decline in egg quantity.

Age and Egg Quality

Age plays a significant role in the quality of a woman's eggs and can have a profound impact on her fertility. As women age, the quality of their eggs naturally declines, making it more difficult to conceive and increasing the risk of chromosomal abnormalities and miscarriages.

With age, the genetic material in a woman's eggs becomes more prone to errors, leading to an increased risk of chromosomal abnormalities such as Down syndrome. This is because as eggs age, they accumulate more genetic mutations, which can affect the development of the embryo and increase the likelihood of miscarriage.

Furthermore, the decline in egg quality with age can also affect the success rates of fertility treatments. Older women may have a lower chance of achieving a successful pregnancy through methods such as in vitro fertilization (IVF) due to the poorer quality of their eggs.

It is important for women to be aware of the impact of age on egg quality and the associated risks. By understanding these factors, women can make informed decisions about their reproductive health and consider options such as fertility preservation or seeking assistance from a fertility specialist.

The Role of AMH

The role of Anti-Mullerian Hormone (AMH) in female fertility is a topic of great interest and importance. AMH is a hormone produced by the cells in the ovaries and serves as a marker for ovarian reserve, which refers to the number and quality of eggs a woman has left. As women age, their ovarian reserve naturally declines, resulting in a decrease in both the quantity and quality of eggs. This decline in ovarian reserve is closely linked to age-related fertility decline. AMH levels can help assess a woman's ovarian reserve and provide valuable information about her fertility potential. A blood test can measure the levels of AMH in a woman's body, and the results can help determine her chances of conceiving naturally or with the help of assisted reproductive technologies. High levels of AMH indicate a good ovarian reserve, while low levels may suggest a diminished reserve. It's important to note that while AMH levels can provide insight into a woman's ovarian reserve, they are not the sole indicator of fertility. Other factors, such as egg quality and overall health, also play a role in determining fertility. In conclusion, AMH plays a crucial role in assessing a woman's ovarian reserve and understanding age-related fertility decline. By measuring AMH levels, healthcare professionals can provide valuable information to women about their fertility potential and guide them in making informed decisions about family planning.

Age and Ovarian Reserve Testing

Age and Ovarian Reserve Testing

Ovarian reserve testing plays a crucial role in assessing a woman's fertility potential and predicting her chances of conceiving. As women age, their ovarian reserve, which refers to the number and quality of eggs remaining in the ovaries, naturally declines. Ovarian reserve testing helps determine the quantity and quality of a woman's eggs, providing valuable insights into her reproductive health.

There are several methods used for ovarian reserve testing, including blood tests and ultrasound examinations. Blood tests measure the levels of certain hormones, such as Anti-Mullerian Hormone (AMH) and Follicle-Stimulating Hormone (FSH), which can indicate the quantity and quality of a woman's eggs. Ultrasound examinations, on the other hand, assess the number of follicles in the ovaries, which can also provide information about ovarian reserve.

By undergoing ovarian reserve testing, women can gain a better understanding of their fertility potential and make informed decisions about family planning. If the results indicate a lower ovarian reserve, it may be an indication that the woman should consider starting a family sooner rather than later. On the other hand, if the results show a healthy ovarian reserve, it can provide reassurance and peace of mind.

It's important to note that while ovarian reserve testing can provide valuable information, it is not a definitive predictor of fertility. It is just one piece of the puzzle and should be considered alongside other factors, such as overall health, lifestyle choices, and any underlying fertility issues. Consulting with a fertility specialist or reproductive endocrinologist is recommended to fully understand the implications of ovarian reserve testing results and to explore the available options for achieving pregnancy.

Age and Menstrual Cycle

Age plays a significant role in the menstrual cycle of a woman. As women age, their menstrual cycles can undergo various changes, including alterations in cycle length, regularity, and ovulation patterns. These changes can have implications for fertility and the ability to conceive.

One of the most noticeable changes in the menstrual cycle with age is the length of the cycle. In younger women, the menstrual cycle typically lasts around 28 days, but as women get older, the cycle length can become shorter or longer. This variation in cycle length can make it more challenging to predict ovulation and determine the most fertile days for conception.

Another change that occurs with age is the irregularity of the menstrual cycle. As women approach perimenopause and menopause, their hormone levels fluctuate, leading to irregular periods. Some months, the menstrual cycle may be longer or shorter than usual, and there may be skipped periods or spotting between periods. These irregularities can make it more difficult to track ovulation and plan for pregnancy.

In addition to changes in cycle length and regularity, age can also affect ovulation patterns. Ovulation is the release of an egg from the ovary, and it typically occurs around the middle of the menstrual cycle. However, as women age, the frequency and regularity of ovulation can decline. This can make it more challenging to conceive, as ovulation is necessary for fertilization to occur.

It is important for women to be aware of these changes in their menstrual cycle as they age, especially if they are trying to conceive. Tracking and monitoring the menstrual cycle can provide valuable information about fertility and help women identify potential issues or irregularities. If a woman is experiencing significant changes or concerns about her menstrual cycle, it is recommended to consult with a healthcare professional who can provide guidance and support.

Age and Reproductive Hormones

Age plays a significant role in the levels of reproductive hormones, including estrogen and progesterone, and their impact on fertility. As women age, their hormone levels naturally fluctuate, which can affect their ability to conceive and have a healthy pregnancy.

Estrogen is a hormone that plays a crucial role in the development and maturation of eggs in the ovaries. As women get older, their estrogen levels start to decline, leading to a decrease in the number and quality of eggs available for fertilization. This decline in egg quantity and quality can make it more difficult for women to get pregnant and increase the risk of pregnancy complications.

Progesterone, on the other hand, is a hormone that prepares the uterus for pregnancy and helps maintain a healthy pregnancy. As women age, their progesterone levels may also decrease, which can affect the implantation of a fertilized egg and increase the risk of miscarriage.

Table 1: Hormonal Changes with Age

Age Range   Estrogen Levels   Progesterone Levels

20-30	High	Stable
30-40	Gradual decline	Slight decline
40-50	Significant decline	Further decline

It is important for women to be aware of these hormonal changes and their potential impact on fertility. If you are trying to conceive and are concerned about your hormone levels, it is recommended to consult with a healthcare provider who specializes in reproductive endocrinology. They can assess your hormone levels through blood tests and provide guidance on fertility treatments or interventions that may be appropriate for your individual situation.

Key Takeaways:

- Age can affect the levels of reproductive hormones, such as estrogen and progesterone.
- Decreased estrogen levels can lead to a decline in the number and quality of eggs.
- Lower progesterone levels can impact the implantation of a fertilized egg and increase the risk of miscarriage.
- Consulting with a reproductive endocrinologist can help assess hormone levels and guide fertility treatment options.

Age and Fertility Treatments

Age can have a significant impact on a woman's fertility, especially as she gets older. For women who are trying to conceive at an older age, there are various fertility treatments available that can help increase their chances of getting pregnant. One such option is assisted reproductive technologies like in vitro fertilization (IVF).

IVF involves the retrieval of eggs from the woman's ovaries, which are then fertilized with sperm in a laboratory. The resulting embryos are then transferred back into the woman's uterus, with the hope of achieving a successful pregnancy. IVF can be a viable option for women who may have age-related fertility challenges, as it bypasses some of the issues associated with age, such as a decrease in egg quantity and quality.

Another fertility treatment option for women trying to conceive at an older age is egg freezing. This procedure involves the retrieval and freezing of a woman's eggs for future use. By freezing their eggs at a younger age, women can preserve their fertility and increase their chances of conception in the future, when they may be ready to start a family.

It's important to note that the success rates of using frozen eggs in fertility treatments can vary depending on various factors, including the woman's age at the time of freezing. Generally, the younger the woman is when she freezes her eggs, the higher the chances of a successful pregnancy using those eggs in the future.

In cases where a woman's own eggs are no longer viable due to age-related factors, the option of using donor eggs may be considered. Donor eggs are typically obtained from younger women who have undergone ovarian stimulation and egg retrieval. These eggs are then fertilized with the recipient's partner's sperm and transferred into the recipient's uterus.

Overall, there are several fertility treatment options available for women who are trying to conceive at an older age. These options can help increase the chances of pregnancy and provide hope for women who may be facing age-related fertility challenges.

In Vitro Fertilization (IVF)

IVF, or In Vitro Fertilization, is a fertility treatment that can be a game-changer for women facing age-related fertility challenges. It offers hope and increased chances of pregnancy, even when natural conception seems unlikely.

During IVF, eggs are retrieved from the woman's ovaries and fertilized with sperm in a laboratory setting. The resulting embryos are then carefully monitored and, once deemed viable, transferred back into the woman's uterus. This process bypasses any potential issues with egg quality or quantity, making it an effective solution for women with age-related fertility decline.

IVF can help overcome age-related fertility challenges in several ways. Firstly, it allows for the use of donor eggs, which can provide healthier and more viable embryos for women who may have diminished egg quality. Additionally, IVF can help overcome issues with low ovarian reserve by

stimulating the ovaries to produce multiple eggs, increasing
the chances of successful fertilization and implantation.

Age-related fertility challenges can be disheartening, but
IVF offers a ray of hope. It provides women with the
opportunity to conceive and have a healthy pregnancy, even
when age may be working against them. By taking
advantage of the advancements in assisted reproductive
technologies, women can increase their chances of
achieving their dream of becoming a mother.

Egg Freezing

Egg freezing has become a popular option for women who
want to preserve their fertility and increase their chances of
conceiving in the future. This technique involves retrieving
a woman's eggs and freezing them for later use. The frozen
eggs can be thawed and fertilized with sperm when the
woman is ready to have a child.

The growing trend of egg freezing can be attributed to
several factors. Firstly, it allows women to extend their
reproductive lifespan, giving them more time to pursue their
personal and professional goals before starting a family. By
freezing their eggs at a younger age, when they are more
likely to have a higher egg quality and quantity, women can
increase their chances of a successful pregnancy later in life.

Egg freezing also provides a sense of security and peace of
mind for women who may be concerned about their future
fertility. It offers them the opportunity to preserve their eggs
before any decline in fertility occurs due to age or other

factors. This can be particularly beneficial for women who have medical conditions that may affect their fertility or those who are planning to undergo treatments that could potentially impact their reproductive health.

It is important to note that the success rates of using frozen eggs vary depending on several factors, including the woman's age at the time of egg freezing. Generally, the younger the woman is when she freezes her eggs, the higher the chances of a successful pregnancy. However, advancements in freezing techniques, such as vitrification, have significantly improved the survival rates of frozen eggs, leading to higher success rates overall.

Egg freezing is a complex process that involves several steps. Firstly, the woman undergoes ovarian stimulation to produce multiple eggs. These eggs are then retrieved through a minimally invasive procedure known as egg retrieval. The retrieved eggs are carefully frozen and stored in a cryopreservation facility until the woman is ready to use them.

When the woman decides to use her frozen eggs, they are thawed and fertilized with sperm through a process called in vitro fertilization (IVF). The resulting embryos are then transferred to the woman's uterus in the hopes of achieving a successful pregnancy.

While egg freezing offers women the opportunity to preserve their fertility, it is important to understand that it is not a guarantee of future pregnancy. The success of using frozen eggs depends on various factors, including the woman's age, overall health, and the quality of the eggs at the time of freezing.

It is recommended that women considering egg freezing consult with a fertility specialist who can provide them with personalized advice and guidance. The specialist can evaluate their individual circumstances and help them make informed decisions about their fertility preservation options.

Success Rates of Frozen Eggs

When it comes to fertility treatments, one option that has gained popularity in recent years is the use of frozen eggs. This innovative technique involves freezing a woman's eggs at a young age when they are still of high quality and can be used in the future when she is ready to conceive.

The success rates of using frozen eggs in fertility treatments can vary depending on several factors, including the age of the woman at the time of egg freezing and the age at which the eggs are thawed and used for fertilization. Generally, younger women who freeze their eggs have higher success rates compared to older women.

Studies have shown that the age at which a woman freezes her eggs plays a significant role in the success of the procedure. The younger the woman, the higher the chances of success. For example, women who freeze their eggs in their early 30s may have a higher likelihood of achieving a successful pregnancy compared to those who freeze their eggs in their late 30s or early 40s.

It's important to note that the success rates of frozen eggs also depend on the quality of the eggs and the overall health of the woman. Factors such as underlying medical conditions, lifestyle choices, and genetic factors can influence the outcome of fertility treatments using frozen eggs.

Additionally, the age at which the frozen eggs are thawed and used for fertilization can impact the success rates. The younger the woman at the time of thawing and fertilization, the higher the chances of a successful pregnancy.

In conclusion, while using frozen eggs in fertility treatments can offer hope to women who wish to preserve their fertility, it's crucial to consider the impact of age on the success rates. Younger women who freeze their eggs at an early age tend to have higher success rates compared to older women. However, individual factors and overall health should also be taken into account when assessing the likelihood of achieving a successful pregnancy using frozen eggs.

Donor Eggs

The option of using donor eggs is available to women who are unable to conceive with their own eggs due to age-related factors. As women age, the number and quality of their eggs naturally decline, making it more difficult to achieve a successful pregnancy. Donor eggs offer a solution by providing healthy and viable eggs from a younger woman.

Using donor eggs involves a process called egg donation, where a young and healthy woman donates her eggs to be used by another woman who is unable to produce viable eggs. This option allows women who have experienced age-related fertility decline to still have the opportunity to conceive and carry a pregnancy to term.

Donor eggs are typically obtained from anonymous donors who have undergone thorough medical and genetic screening to ensure the highest chances of success. The eggs are then fertilized with the intended father's sperm or donor sperm through a procedure called in vitro fertilization (IVF).

After fertilization, the resulting embryos are transferred into the recipient's uterus, where they can implant and develop into a pregnancy. Donor egg IVF has shown high success rates, as the quality of the donor eggs is typically excellent.

It is important for women considering the option of donor eggs to carefully consider the emotional and ethical implications of this choice. While it provides a viable path to parenthood, it may involve complex emotions and considerations. Seeking professional guidance and support throughout the process is highly recommended.

Age and Pregnancy Risks

Age plays a significant role in the risks and complications associated with pregnancy. As women get older, their chances of experiencing certain health issues during pregnancy increase. It is important for women to be aware of these risks and take necessary precautions.

One of the common risks associated with pregnancy at an older age is gestational diabetes. This condition occurs when a woman's body cannot produce enough insulin to regulate blood sugar levels during pregnancy. Women who develop gestational diabetes are at a higher risk of developing type 2 diabetes later in life. Regular monitoring of blood sugar levels and following a healthy diet can help manage gestational diabetes.

High blood pressure, or hypertension, is another risk that is more prevalent in older pregnant women. High blood pressure can lead to complications such as preeclampsia, a condition characterized by high blood pressure and damage to organs such as the liver and kidneys. Regular prenatal check-ups and monitoring blood pressure levels are essential to manage and prevent complications associated with high blood pressure.

Genetic disorders are also more common in pregnancies at an older age. The risk of chromosomal abnormalities, such as Down syndrome, increases as a woman's age advances. Genetic counseling and prenatal testing can help identify any potential genetic disorders early on and allow parents to make informed decisions about their pregnancy.

It is important for women considering pregnancy at an older age to discuss these risks with their healthcare provider. Together, they can develop a personalized plan to monitor and manage any potential complications. By staying informed and taking proactive measures, women can increase their chances of having a healthy pregnancy and a successful outcome.

Age and Miscarriage

The risk of miscarriage increases significantly in women of advanced maternal age. Advanced maternal age is generally considered to be 35 years and older. Several factors contribute to this increased risk, including:

- Decreased egg quality: As women age, the quality of their eggs declines. This can lead to chromosomal abnormalities in the embryo, making it less likely to develop into a healthy pregnancy.
- Decreased egg quantity: Women are born with a finite number of eggs, and as they age, the number of eggs decreases. This can reduce the chances of a successful pregnancy and increase the risk of miscarriage.
- Increased risk of underlying health conditions: Older women may have a higher prevalence of underlying health conditions, such as diabetes or high blood pressure. These conditions can increase the risk of miscarriage.
- Uterine abnormalities: Age can also be associated with changes in the uterus, such as fibroids or polyps, which can interfere with implantation and increase the risk of miscarriage.

It is important for women of advanced maternal age to be aware of these factors and seek appropriate medical care and support during pregnancy. Regular prenatal care and monitoring can help identify any potential issues early on and improve the chances of a successful pregnancy.

Age and Birth Defects

The correlation between maternal age and the incidence of birth defects, including Down syndrome and other chromosomal abnormalities.

As women age, the risk of giving birth to a baby with birth defects increases. One of the most well-known birth defects associated with advanced maternal age is Down syndrome. Down syndrome is a genetic condition that occurs when there is an extra copy of chromosome 21. The likelihood of having a baby with Down syndrome increases significantly as a woman gets older.

In addition to Down syndrome, there is also an increased risk of other chromosomal abnormalities, such as trisomy 18 and trisomy 13, as well as structural birth defects. These structural birth defects can affect various parts of the baby's body, including the heart, brain, and limbs.

The exact reasons behind the increased risk of birth defects with age are not fully understood. However, it is believed that the quality of a woman's eggs may play a role. As women age, the quality of their eggs decreases, which can lead to an increased risk of chromosomal abnormalities and other genetic defects in the developing fetus.

Prenatal testing and screening are important tools for identifying potential birth defects and helping women make informed decisions about their pregnancy. Tests such as amniocentesis and chorionic villus sampling (CVS) can detect chromosomal abnormalities, while ultrasound scans can identify certain structural birth defects.

It is important for women of advanced maternal age to discuss their options with their healthcare provider and consider the potential risks and benefits of prenatal testing. This information can help them make decisions about their pregnancy and ensure they receive appropriate care and support throughout the process.

Prenatal Testing and Screening

The importance of prenatal testing and screening for older women cannot be overstated. As women age, the risk of genetic disorders and chromosomal abnormalities in their offspring increases. Prenatal testing and screening allow these women to assess the risk and make informed decisions about their pregnancy.

Prenatal testing typically involves a combination of blood tests, ultrasounds, and genetic screening. These tests can detect various genetic disorders, such as Down syndrome and other chromosomal abnormalities. By identifying these conditions early on, women have the opportunity to consult with healthcare professionals and specialists, understand the potential implications, and consider their options.

Screening tests, such as non-invasive prenatal testing (NIPT), can provide valuable information about the likelihood of certain genetic conditions. NIPT analyzes fetal DNA in the mother's blood and can detect conditions like Down syndrome with a high degree of accuracy. However, it's important to note that NIPT is a screening test and not a diagnostic test. If the results indicate a higher risk, further diagnostic tests, such as amniocentesis or chorionic villus sampling (CVS), may be recommended to confirm the diagnosis.

Prenatal testing and screening also offer peace of mind for older women who may be concerned about the health of their baby. It allows them to proactively manage any potential risks and make decisions that are best for themselves and their families. It's important for women to discuss their options and preferences with their healthcare providers to determine the most appropriate testing and screening approach for their individual circumstances.

Age and Fertility Preservation

As women choose to delay childbearing for various reasons, fertility preservation options have become increasingly important. Fertility preservation allows women to freeze their eggs or embryos at a younger age, preserving their fertility potential for the future. Two common methods of fertility preservation are egg freezing and embryo cryopreservation.

Egg Freezing:

Egg freezing, also known as oocyte cryopreservation, involves extracting a woman's eggs and freezing them for later use. This process allows women to preserve their eggs at a younger age when they are more likely to be of higher quality and have a better chance of resulting in a successful pregnancy. When a woman is ready to conceive, the frozen eggs can be thawed, fertilized with sperm, and implanted into the uterus through in vitro fertilization (IVF).

Egg freezing offers women the flexibility to pursue their career, education, or personal goals without the worry of age-related decline in fertility. It provides a sense of control over their reproductive timeline, giving them the opportunity to have biological children when they are ready.

Embryo Cryopreservation:

Embryo cryopreservation involves the fertilization of a woman's eggs with sperm to create embryos, which are then frozen for future use. This method is often used by couples undergoing IVF who have surplus embryos that are not immediately transferred to the woman's uterus. By freezing these embryos, they can be stored and used in subsequent IVF cycles, allowing the couple to try for pregnancy at a later time.

Embryo cryopreservation is particularly beneficial for couples who have concerns about the quality or quantity of the woman's eggs, as it allows them to preserve viable embryos for future use. It also offers the possibility of using donor sperm or eggs, giving couples more options in their journey to parenthood.

Fertility preservation through egg freezing and embryo cryopreservation has revolutionized the field of reproductive medicine, providing hope and options for women who wish to delay childbearing. These methods offer a chance to overcome the age-related decline in fertility and increase the likelihood of a successful pregnancy when the time is right.

Egg Freezing

Egg freezing, also known as oocyte cryopreservation, is a process that allows women to preserve their fertility by freezing their eggs for future use. This procedure involves stimulating the ovaries to produce multiple eggs, which are then retrieved and frozen for later use. The frozen eggs can be stored for several years, maintaining their quality and viability.

Egg freezing offers several potential benefits for women who want to preserve their fertility. Firstly, it provides an option for women who may not be ready to start a family yet but want to ensure that they have the possibility in the future. This is particularly relevant for women who are focused on their careers, pursuing higher education, or have not found a suitable partner.

Additionally, egg freezing can be beneficial for women who are facing medical treatments that may affect their fertility, such as chemotherapy or radiation therapy. By freezing their eggs before undergoing these treatments, women can increase their chances of conceiving later on, even if their fertility is compromised by the treatment.

Success rates of egg freezing have improved significantly in recent years, thanks to advances in cryopreservation techniques. The success of the procedure depends on various factors, including the woman's age at the time of egg freezing. Generally, the younger the woman, the higher the chances of success, as younger eggs tend to have better quality and higher chances of fertilization.

It's important to note that while egg freezing can offer a viable option for preserving fertility, it does not guarantee a successful pregnancy in the future. The success rates vary depending on individual factors and the quality of the eggs at the time of freezing. Therefore, it's advisable for women considering egg freezing to consult with a fertility specialist who can provide personalized guidance and information about their specific circumstances.

Embryo Cryopreservation

Embryo cryopreservation is a revolutionary technique that offers women a viable option to preserve their fertility and increase their chances of conceiving in the future. This process involves freezing and storing embryos, which are fertilized eggs, for later use in assisted reproductive technologies like in vitro fertilization (IVF).

Embryo cryopreservation begins with the stimulation of a woman's ovaries to produce multiple eggs. These eggs are then retrieved and fertilized with sperm in a laboratory setting. The resulting embryos are carefully monitored and evaluated for quality before being frozen using a technique called vitrification. Vitrification ensures that the embryos are preserved at extremely low temperatures without any damage to their structure or viability.

By freezing embryos, women can preserve their fertility at a specific point in time when their eggs are still healthy and of good quality. This is particularly beneficial for women who may face age-related fertility decline or those who are undergoing medical treatments that may affect their reproductive health, such as chemotherapy or radiation therapy.

Embryo cryopreservation also offers women the flexibility to plan their pregnancies according to their life circumstances. They can choose to delay childbearing for personal or professional reasons, knowing that their frozen embryos are safely stored and available for future use.

When a woman is ready to conceive, the frozen embryos can be thawed and transferred to her uterus during an IVF procedure. The success rates of embryo cryopreservation have significantly improved over the years, with high chances of achieving a successful pregnancy.

It is important to note that embryo cryopreservation may not be suitable for every woman, as it requires the initial step of undergoing IVF treatment to create the embryos. Additionally, there may be ethical and personal considerations involved in deciding to freeze and use embryos. It is essential for women to consult with fertility specialists and consider their individual circumstances before opting for embryo cryopreservation.

Age and Emotional Considerations

Age can bring about a range of emotional considerations when it comes to fertility. Many women feel the pressure to conceive as they get older, especially if they have not yet started a family. Society often places expectations on women to have children at a certain age, which can create feelings of anxiety and stress. It's important for women to remember that everyone's journey is unique, and there is no one-size-fits-all timeline for starting a family.

Coping with infertility can also be emotionally challenging. When a woman is unable to conceive naturally or experiences difficulties in getting pregnant, it can lead to feelings of frustration, sadness, and even grief. It's important for women to seek support during this time, whether it's through talking to a trusted friend or family member, joining a support group, or seeking professional counseling. Having a strong support system can help women navigate the emotional ups and downs of infertility and provide a safe space to express their feelings.

Exploring alternative paths to parenthood is another important aspect to consider. For some women, conceiving naturally may not be possible, and they may need to explore options such as adoption, surrogacy, or fostering. These alternative paths can offer a fulfilling and rewarding way to become a parent and create a loving family. However, it's essential to understand the legal and ethical considerations involved in these options and seek professional guidance to ensure a smooth and informed decision-making process.

Overall, addressing the emotional aspects of fertility and age is crucial for women who are navigating the journey of starting a family. It's important to acknowledge and validate the range of emotions that can arise, from the pressure to conceive to the challenges of coping with infertility. Seeking support, exploring alternative paths to parenthood, and taking care of one's emotional well-being are all essential steps in this process.

Emotional Impact of Age-Related Infertility

The emotional impact of age-related infertility can be significant and challenging for women. As they struggle to conceive and face the realization that their biological clock is ticking, it is common for feelings of sadness, frustration, and even guilt to arise. The desire to have a child is deeply ingrained in many women, and the inability to fulfill this desire can lead to a range of emotions.

One of the main emotional challenges faced by women dealing with age-related infertility is the pressure they feel from society, family, and even themselves. There is often an expectation that women should be able to conceive naturally and easily, and when this does not happen, it can be incredibly disheartening. Women may feel like they have failed or that there is something wrong with them.

It is important for women facing age-related infertility to seek support and understanding. Talking to a therapist or joining a support group can provide a safe space to express emotions and share experiences with others who are going through similar challenges. These support systems can offer validation, empathy, and guidance on coping strategies.

Alternative Paths to Parenthood

For women who are unable to conceive naturally, there are alternative paths to parenthood that can fulfill their desire to have a child. These options include adoption, surrogacy, and fostering. Each of these alternatives offers unique opportunities and considerations, allowing women to create a loving and nurturing family.

Adoption: Adoption is a beautiful way to build a family and provide a loving home for a child in need. Whether through domestic or international adoption, women can welcome a child into their lives and provide them with a stable and supportive environment. The adoption process involves legal procedures and assessments to ensure the well-being of both the child and the adopting parents.

Surrogacy: Surrogacy involves another woman carrying a pregnancy on behalf of the intended parents. This option is suitable for women who are unable to carry a pregnancy themselves due to medical reasons or infertility. In surrogacy, the intended parents work closely with a surrogate mother, who carries the pregnancy and gives birth to the child. Legal agreements and medical procedures are involved to ensure the rights and responsibilities of all parties involved.

Fostering: Fostering provides a temporary home for children who are in need of care and support. Women who are unable to conceive naturally can open their hearts and homes to foster children, providing them with a safe and nurturing environment. Fostering allows women to make a difference in a child's life while also experiencing the joys and challenges of parenthood.

When considering alternative paths to parenthood, it is important for women to carefully evaluate their options and seek professional guidance. Legal and ethical considerations play a significant role in these alternative paths, and it is essential to navigate the process with the assistance of knowledgeable professionals.

- Adoption provides a loving home for a child in need.
- Surrogacy involves another woman carrying a pregnancy on behalf of the intended parents.
- Fostering provides a temporary home for children who are in need of care and support.

Legal and Ethical Considerations

When exploring alternative paths to parenthood, it is crucial to consider the legal and ethical considerations that come into play. Each option, whether it be adoption, surrogacy, or fostering, has its own set of rules and regulations that must be followed to ensure a smooth and legal process.

Adoption, for example, requires prospective parents to meet certain criteria and go through a thorough screening process to ensure they are fit to provide a loving and stable home for a child. It is important to understand the legal requirements and procedures involved in adoption and seek professional guidance to navigate through the complexities of the adoption process.

Surrogacy, on the other hand, involves a surrogate mother carrying a child on behalf of the intended parents. This can raise various legal and ethical considerations, such as the rights and responsibilities of all parties involved, the legality of surrogacy agreements in different jurisdictions, and the potential emotional and psychological impact on all parties. Seeking legal advice and guidance from professionals experienced in surrogacy laws is crucial to ensure a smooth and ethical surrogacy journey.

Fostering is another alternative path to parenthood that requires careful consideration of legal and ethical aspects. Fostering involves providing a temporary home for a child who is unable to live with their birth parents. The process of becoming a foster parent involves background checks, home visits, and training to ensure the safety and well-being of the child. Understanding the legal rights and responsibilities of foster parents and seeking professional guidance can help navigate the complexities of the fostering system.

In all alternative paths to parenthood, seeking professional guidance is of utmost importance. Professionals such as lawyers, adoption agencies, surrogacy agencies, and social workers specialize in the legal and ethical aspects of these processes. They can provide valuable advice, support, and guidance to ensure that the chosen path is legally compliant, ethical, and in the best interest of all parties involved.

Support and Counseling

The emotional journey of fertility and age-related challenges can be overwhelming for women. It is essential to have a support system in place to help navigate through these difficult times. Support groups, counseling, and therapy play a crucial role in providing the necessary emotional support and guidance.

Support groups offer a safe space for women to share their experiences, fears, and frustrations with others who are going through similar situations. Being surrounded by individuals who understand the emotional rollercoaster of fertility struggles can provide a sense of belonging and validation. These groups often offer valuable resources, information, and coping strategies to help women cope with the challenges they face.

Counseling and therapy can be beneficial for women dealing with fertility and age-related issues. A trained therapist or counselor can provide a non-judgmental and supportive environment where women can explore their feelings, fears, and concerns. They can help women develop coping mechanisms, manage stress, and navigate the complex emotions that come with fertility struggles.

Therapy sessions may involve individual counseling or couples counseling, depending on the specific needs and circumstances. Couples counseling can help partners communicate effectively, manage conflicts, and support each other through the ups and downs of the fertility journey.

It is important to seek professional help from licensed therapists or counselors who specialize in fertility and reproductive health. They have the expertise and knowledge to address the unique challenges that women face during this time. Additionally, they can provide guidance on alternative paths to parenthood, such as adoption or surrogacy, if natural conception is not possible.

Remember, seeking support and counseling is not a sign of weakness but a proactive step towards emotional well-being. It is crucial to prioritize self-care and surround yourself with a supportive network of professionals and loved ones who can provide the necessary guidance and understanding.

Frequently Asked Questions

- **1. How does age affect female fertility?**

  As women age, their fertility naturally declines. This is because the number and quality of eggs decrease over time. Additionally, there is an increased risk of pregnancy complications.

- **2. What is the role of Anti-Mullerian Hormone (AMH) in fertility?**

AMH is a hormone that serves as a marker for ovarian reserve. It helps assess a woman's fertility potential and is closely correlated with age-related fertility decline.

- **3. How does age impact egg quantity?**

A woman's egg quantity decreases as she gets older. This means that she has fewer eggs available for fertilization, which can reduce her chances of getting pregnant.

- **4. What is the effect of age on egg quality?**

Age can negatively affect the quality of a woman's eggs. Older eggs are more likely to have chromosomal abnormalities, leading to an increased risk of miscarriages and birth defects.

- **5. Can fertility treatments help overcome age-related challenges?**

Yes, there are fertility treatments available, such as In Vitro Fertilization (IVF), that can help women overcome age-related fertility challenges and increase their chances of getting pregnant.

- **6. What is egg freezing and how can it benefit women?**

Egg freezing is a process where a woman's eggs are preserved for future use. It can benefit women who want to delay childbearing, as it allows them to use their frozen eggs later when they are ready to conceive.

- ## 7. What are the success rates of using frozen eggs in fertility treatments?

  The success rates of using frozen eggs in fertility treatments can vary depending on various factors, including the woman's age at the time of egg freezing. Generally, younger women tend to have higher success rates.

- ## 8. Is using donor eggs an option for women with age-related fertility issues?

  Yes, using donor eggs can be an option for women who are unable to conceive with their own eggs due to age-related factors. This allows them to still experience pregnancy and have a child.

- ## 9. What are the increased risks associated with pregnancy at an older age?

  Pregnancy at an older age carries higher risks, including gestational diabetes, high blood pressure, and an increased chance of genetic disorders in the baby.

- ## 10. How can women cope with the emotional challenges of age-related infertility?

Dealing with age-related infertility can be emotionally challenging. Seeking support from support groups, counseling, and therapy can help women navigate this journey and find emotional well-being.

Have Questions / Comments?

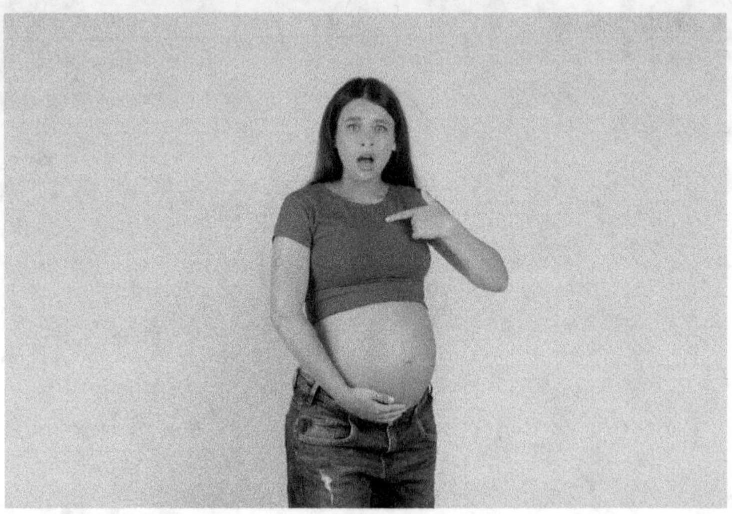

This book was designed to cover as much info as possible but I know I have probably missed something, or some new amazing discovery that has just come out.

If you notice something missing or have a question that I failed to answer, please get in touch and let me know. If I can, I will email you an answer and also update the book so others can also benefit from it.

Thanks For Being Awesome :)

Submit Your Questions / Comments At:

Get In Touch at Babydreamers.net

Get How To Be A Super Mom - 100% FREE

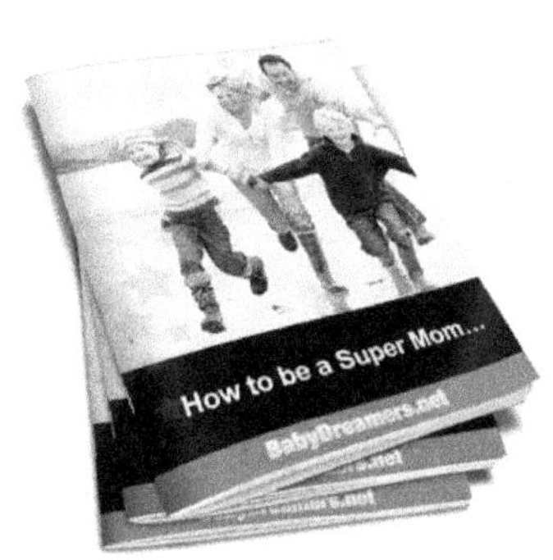

For being one of our amazing readers, we would love to offer you another book we have created, 100% free.

Being a mom is probably the most important job in the world – we've all heard that, and it's true. You're bringing up the next generation of wonderful, intelligent, loving, creative, responsible people.

We all want to be Super Mom and to be everything and do everything, but it this possible?

Being a Super Mom is possible, but you have to learn how to empower yourself to be the kind of Super Mom that you feel you need to be, keeping in mind that the title Super Mom doesn't mean the same thing to everyone.

Get How to be a Super Mom For Free at

BabyDreamers.net

www.ingramcontent.com/pod-product-compliance
Lightning Source LLC
Chambersburg PA
CBHW071006260726

48661CB00007B/2816